HOW TO KEEP THE PAUSE OUT OF ANDROPAUSE

Men at midlife and beyond can maintain their sexual fitness, interest, and vitality in spite of the ravages of the normal aging process. Physical and psychological issues that affect sexual response can be prevented and/or treated with this multifaceted, integrative approach. Strategies that you might not associate with sexual function such as brain mapping, blood testing, noninvasive ultrasound techniques, psychological evaluation, and nutritional and medicinal supplementation can lead you to enhanced sexual wellness.

Eric Braverman, M.D., is the Director of the Place for Achieving Total Health (PATH Medical), with locations in New York City, and Penndel, Pennsylvania, and a national network of affiliated medical practices. Dr. Braverman received his B.A. summa-cum-laude from Brandeis University and his M.D. with honors from New York University Medical School, after which he did postgraduate work in Internal Medicine with a Yale Medical School affiliate in Greenwich, Connecticut.

Dr. Braverman's current pursuits include private practice at all PATH Medical sites as well as directorship of the PATH Foundation, a nonprofit research organization established to collect information concerning the diagnosis, prevention, and treatment of all aspects of brain chemical disorders, with specific focus on the impact of brain illness on overall health. PATH Foundation work is conducted with the affiliated associates; collaborative projects have yielded revolutionary research documenting that brain disease or genetic weaknesses significantly contribute to psychiatric disorders. The PATH Foundation also has been intensely involved in the development of the usage of both clinic-use and at-home therapies dedicated to improving the health of the brain.

Dr. Braverman has published over eighty research papers with many colleagues. He has also published books for the health-conscious general readership, including, in conjunction with Dr. Carl C. Pfeiffer, *Zinc and Other Micro-Nutrients;* *The Healing Nutrients Within, 2nd ed.* with Drs. Pfeiffer, Blum, and Smayda; and *The PATH Wellness Manual* (see Further Reading).

Male Sexual Fitness

Causes and Solutions for Andropause

by Eric R. Braverman, M.D.

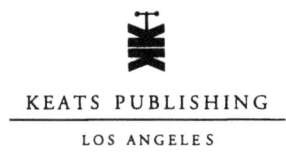

KEATS PUBLISHING

LOS ANGELES

NTC/Contemporary Publishing Group

The author wishes to make the following acknowledgments:

- To Catherine Cebula, whose research, writing, and editorial talent made this guide possible.
- To Richard Smayda, D.O., whose input and insights enhanced this guide.
- To the PATH Medical team, whose professionalism and combined abilities ensure a prompt and successful healing process for all of our patients.

Male Sexual Fitness is intended solely for informational and educational purposes and not as medical advice. Please consult a health care professional if you have questions about your health.

MALE SEXUAL FITNESS: CAUSES AND SOLUTIONS FOR ANDROPAUSE

Contents

Introduction 6
Normal Sexual Response Cycle.. 12
Andropause (Male Menopause) 13
Brain State: Physical and Psychological Health.................. 15
Circulatory Issues 21
Hormones.. 25
Beneficial Options That May Help in Regaining
    Sexual Vitality 33
Additional Important Medical Issues for Sexual Fitness.. 37
Environmental Issues.. 43
Other Approaches 45
Conclusion... 47
Glossary 48
Further Reading.. 49
Resources... 50
Bibliography.. 52

Many men at midlife and beyond are increasingly concerned with their outward appearance: They exercise to firm muscles or achieve leaner body mass; they attempt various topical and oral agents to retain a full head of hair or keep their skin smooth. These men ought to be equally concerned with monitoring and maintaining their sexual health and vitality.

You will benefit from reading this guide if you are:

- a man who already follows basic guidelines for good health (as specified by your physician);
- a companion to a man who presently addresses his basic physical needs;
- a man who has noticed some symptoms of waning sexual fitness; or
- a man's companion who has noticed a decline in your partner's sexual health.

AUTHOR'S NOTE CONCERNING VASOCONGESTING AGENTS

In the clinical experience of this author, the sudden and widespread popularity of the class of vasocongesting medications (including Viagra® and Vasomax®) will fade, as more people realize that many cases of sexual dysfunction result from medical issues other than penile circulatory disorder. Viagra, like its natural counterpart the amino acid arginine, promotes enhanced blood flow to the penis. The penis enlarges because Viagra promotes the release of nitric oxide. In essence, an erection is similar to a dose of laughing gas inside an appendage.

Brain state, circulatory state, endocrine state, and neurological state (specifically, of the penis) are all important contributors to male sexuality. Vasocongesting agents do not correct for medical origins of sexual dysfunction caused by common conditions, including:

- chronic anxiety, linked to premature ejaculation
- hormonal deficits, since hormones are essential for sexual health
- damaged nerves (as with diabetics)—intramuscular B12, growth hormone, acetyl carnitine
- chronic medical conditions or altered nutritional state

Vasocongesting agents will continue to be important contributors to the recovery of sexual function in men with vasculature conditions that affect penile blood flow. Recently, one of my patients, a smoker, with a reduced penile blood pressure (assessed by Doppler ultrasound), responded tremendously to Viagra. In such cases as these, vasocongesting medications hold great promise.

In any case of loss of libido or impotence, it is incumbent upon the physician to seek the underlying cause of the patient's dysfunction. This book will demonstrate that because circulatory disorders comprise a small contributing factor in many cases of sexual dysfunction, a limited number of men will respond to vasocongesting medication. In reading this book, you will discover that a great range of medical conditions, the majority of which are easily corrected, contribute to a decline in male sexual fitness.

SEXUAL FITNESS RISK FACTORS

We all know that smoking, drinking, and a sedentary lifestyle—behaviors that can be changed—are risk factors for a heart attack. We are also aware that there are certain genetic factors beyond our control that contribute to risk. So it is with declining sexual function, but the public is less familiar with these factors and not as likely to identify declining sexual function in such terms. However, it is important to do so. Table 1 displays the array of symptoms and conditions frequently associated with loss of sexual function. These factors affect sexual fitness to varying degrees. To estimate your sexual fitness using the risk factors in Table 1, follow these instructions:

1. Check the box next to each symptom or condition which applies to your case. Note that each entry has a number following it; the higher the number, the greater the risk factor, that is, the extent to which it adversely affects sexual fitness.

2. Tabulate your total sexual fitness risk: Add up the values for the boxes that you have checked. Notice that everyone starts with four points of risk, since environmental factors are nearly inescapable (see Environmental Issues).

3. Consult Table 2 to estimate your sexual fitness.

The sooner a man addresses each problem, the more likely he is to recover sexual prowess. Early detection allows prompt intervention and the opportunity to restore sexual vitality.

Table 1.
Checklist of Factors Contributing to Ailing Sexual Fitness

Sexual Indicators of Andropause

Desire/Arousal	Response	Orgasm	Resolution
☐ Decreased desire [1]	☐ Slower time to erection [1]	☐ Difficult or unable to maintain erection through mutual completion of experience [2]	☐ Rapid detumescence (return to flaccid state) [2]
☐ Absence of sexual fantasies [1]	☐ Decreased penile sensitivity [2] ☐ Erections less rigid; shorter duration [2] ☐ Erectile response requires stimulation from partner [1]	☐ Lack of subjective sense of satisfaction [2]	

Overall Physical Condition

- ☐ Hormone imbalances [5]
- ☐ Cardiovascular illnesses [5]
- ☐ Circulatory system issues [5]
- ☐ Penile health, less than ideal [5]

- ☐ Prostate condition [5]
- ☐ Obesity [4]
- ☐ Diabetes mellitus [4]
- ☐ Long-term usage or multiple use of prescription or over-the-counter drugs or both [4]

- ☐ Alcohol or drug abuse [5]
- ☐ Neuropathies [5]
- ☐ Brain injury or malfunction [5]
- ☐ Amino acid imbalances [2]

- ☐ Chronic pain [4]
- ☐ Spinal cord injury [5]
- ☐ Pelvic or urological surgery [3]
- ☐ Free radical damage [2]

- ☒ Environmental exposures [4]

Psychological Conditions

- ☐ Anxiety [5]
- ☐ Attention disorder [5]
- ☐ Maladaptive personality traits [5]
- ☐ Interpersonal skills requiring improvement [4]

Source: Developed at PATH Medical

Table 2.
Estimation of Risk Based on Total Calculation of Factors

Total: Sexual Fitness Risk	Condition of Sexual Fitness
1 to 6	Possibly experiencing early signs of ailing sexual health.
7 to 12	Suboptimal sexual health.
13 and more	Sexual health in jeopardy, prolonged loss of libido likely.

THE SEXUAL CHECKUP

There are several medical conditions which can affect a man's desire, his ability to become aroused and sustain arousal, and to complete the act of sexual intercourse. Many factors contribute to overall sexual wellness. There are four primary body functions to which the underlying origin of lost libido and ailing sexual function may be attributed:

- Brain state
- Circulatory state
- Endocrine state
- Neurological state (specifically, of the penis)

Specific and additional evaluation may be appropriate if a man has a medical condition that complicates his overall health, such as a prostate condition, obesity, or a chronic ailment.

THE SEXUAL TUNE-UP

After proper diagnosis, men will likely regain sexual function once an appropriate, comprehensive treatment is formulated. There are several key elements to the recovery of sexual function:

- Correction of brain physical and psychological issues
- Improvement in circulation and cardiovascular conditions
- Balancing hormone levels—especially deficits

- Nutritional supplementation
- Assisting the function of the penis to achieve and sustain erection.

FOLKLORE VERSUS FACT

The word "testes" comes from the Latin for *witness*, literally meaning that the word of a man was as good as his genitalia. In folklore, the penis symbolizes fertility, power, and aggression. The perception that bigger is better still dominates the image of male sexuality. However, surveys find that women do not consider the size of the penis to be a predominant factor in the sexual experience. Today's women consider arousal stimuli—such as touching and intimate caressing—as invaluable to their definition of "good sex."

Sexually active, intact couples can maintain satisfying sexual lives well into old age. Even if intercourse is problematic due to physical infirmity, intimacy that is satisfying to the participants is possible. Sexuality is not contraindicated due to aging; folklore that suggests this diminishing attractiveness and attraction is, quite simply, inaccurate.

Folklore also says that certain foods have aphrodisiac effects—the ability to arouse or stimulate sexual desire. Foods with seeds, such as strawberries and papayas, have become symbols of fertility; there is even the "passionfruit." Old wives' tales recommend soups of chicken giblets, testicles, and ovaries to promote sexual interest. In earlier times, plants resembling the human shape, such as ginseng and mandrakes, were associated with magical powers in Oriental fables and Biblical tales. These tales have secured a place in beliefs concerning male fertility. None are clinically valid; however, they do attest to the ingrained preoccupation of society with the state of sexual fitness. Flavors of foods or scents of flowers have been suggested as agents to enhance arousal; their action more likely originates from the ability to calm and soothe, leading to bolstered self-confidence, rather than to outright sexual enhancement.

PHASES

The cycle of human sexual response consists of four phases.

Desire

The first phase consists of fantasies and the wish to engage in sexual activity. This reaction is psychological in origin and is enhanced by androgens in men.

Arousal

The second phase consists of a number of physiological changes, plus the subjective sense of sexual pleasure. Arousal depends upon neurological stimulation through the pathways from the spinal cord and the brain, as well as from blood supply. In both sexes, there is an increased heart rate, more rapid breathing, and development of muscular tension throughout the body—most pronounced in the pelvic area and thighs. For both sexes, the major physiological change is vasocongestion (increased blood flow) in the genital area. For women, the manifestations of vasocongestion are vaginal lubrication and swelling of the external genitalia. For men, three main activities inside the penis cause erection (also termed *tumescence*): (1) the helicine arteries receive increased blood flow; (2) the primary mass of the penis—spongy tissue—engorges (fills with blood); (3) the spongy tissue pushes against the outer casing of fibrous sheath. Additionally, the scrotal muscle tightens and the testes elevate: this is the manner in which the body adjusts the angle of the penis for entry into the woman's anatomy.

Orgasm

The third phase is orgasm. Subjectively, for both sexes, orgasm is the peaking of sexual pleasure accompanied by a sense of release from sexual tension. In men, after the semen is produced, it is ejaculated from the penis.

Resolution

The fourth phase is resolution and is accompanied by a sense of pleasure, warmth, well-being, and relaxation. Physiologically, there is a gradual return of heart rate, breathing rate, and muscle tension to the baseline state.

ANDROPAUSE (MALE MENOPAUSE)

Andropause or "male menopause" is a medical condition that may be thought of as the counterpart to menopause in women. In both sexes, the condition is caused by a decline in the levels of hormones related to sexuality and occurs over a period of time: it may begin between the ages of twenty and fifty. Andropause is due to a decrease in testosterone, a type of androgen (a set of hormones that causes the secondary sex characteristics such as facial hair, deepening of voice, and increase in muscle bulk). Male menopause differs from female menopause in three ways:

1. Andropause has a gradual onset. As a result, symptoms are often unrecognized as indicators of declining sexual health. The majority of men will experience a mild rate of decline in free (active) testosterone.

2. Men will continue to release sperm and hence be able to reproduce over a greater period of life.

3. Many medical practitioners consider andropause to be synonymous with *hypogonadism*. However, published research literature contains contradictory conclusions and speculations. We find that hypogonadism is a specific subtype of andropause, so we contend that andro-

pause is a condition that affects the sexual fitness of every man.

PROTOCOLS FOR SEXUAL FITNESS

We have developed a protocol that enables a quick and reliable diagnosis for most cases of male menopause. By doing so, we can place our patients on a customized treatment plan to address the cause(s) of their lost sexual vitality. Table 3 lists the major factors that we have found to be most prevalent in ailing sexual fitness and possible techniques for treatment.

Table 3.
Protocol for Diagnosis and Treatment

Diagnosis	Treatment
Anxiety, depression, stress: Test of Variables of Attention	Medications and supplements to relieve anxiety
Personality profiles: including Millon and Myers-Briggs	Personality de-stressing exercises
Circulatory abnormalities, including penile function: Doppler	Chelation, biofeedback, exercise; creams and inserts (noninvasive erection producing agents)
Endocrine profile, including testosterone, DHEA, growth hormone	Hormone supplementation
Neuropathies: NCVs	Circulatory enhancement agents and exercises

Source: Developed at PATH Medical

We have found that ailing sexual fitness is frequently due to imbalances in the brain. In some cases, the physical brain state—particularly neurotransmission or brain wave malfunctions—affects the patient's health. More often, psychological factors are the source of the problem.

PHYSICAL HEALTH

Electroencephalography (EEG) is a useful tool to evaluate the physical brain state. It can detect physical abnormalities that directly produce illnesses such as epilepsy, migraines or chronic headaches, head trauma, lesions, or cerebrovascular disease. EEG is also useful for enhancing our insight about psychiatric disorders, which often originate with a physical disorder in the brain left undetected except via EEG. Studies also show that asymmetric EEG patterns correlate directly with dysfunctional responses to visual and/or auditory stimuli. In psychological test situations, there are significant differences between normal and dysfunctional subjects in terms of the cognitive activity that occurs within the right temporal area of the brain. When asked to respond to erotic stimuli, the dysfunctional testers responded only to auditory, not visual, stimuli.

Brain Electrical Activity Mapping (BEAM) is a novel and reliable method which extends the concept of computerized EEG monitoring by combining it with deliberately generated auditory or visual stimuli designed to evoke cortical responses. These responses are analyzed for deviance from a set of pre-established normal values; combined with a review of the EEG, the physician may determine medical issues such as:

- physical or psychiatric abnormalities in the brain
- brain wave abnormalities caused by usage of prescription medications, illicit drugs, steroids
- behavioral ailments, such as attention-deficit disorder (ADD), obsessive-compulsive disorder (OCD)
- verbal- or audio-processing impairments

Any of these conditions indicate problems with the conscious mind; thus, detected abnormalities may cause a range of disorders in overall health, such as:

- irritability, hyperactivity, depression, compulsions, unreal thoughts
- overconcentration or lack of focus
- memory loss
- rage or aggression
- difficulty in ability to communicate

Any one of these symptoms, much less a combination of several, may contribute to a lack of sexual desire and unresponsiveness to arousal.

PSYCHOGENIC FACTORS

At the present time, it is largely accepted that the majority of sexual disorders have an organic (physical) basis, rather than a psychological origin (strictly related to the behavior process). Sexual dysfunction can be traced to mechanisms of endocrine physiology as well as to the cellular level, with recent discoveries implicating cellular receptor activity. Physical conditions and drugs can interrupt normal sexual function and add to the majority opinion that, in most cases, physiological factors outweigh psychological ones.

However, if assessment for an organic etiology does not yield a convincing diagnosis, or a trial of one or more medications does not remedy the situation, a psychogenic basis should be assumed. This is a situation where the illness originates in the processes of mental, behavioral, or personality development (or some combination of these factors), but manifests as physical symptoms, and potentially, as sexual dysfunction. To verify such a diagnosis, a physician will conduct an in-depth consultation with the afflicted individual, perhaps with him and his partner together, while utilizing psychological testing.

Sexual dysfunction of a psychogenic basis is variable. It may develop after a period of normal function, or it may be prolonged. The problem may occur with all partners, be limited to previous partners and therefore be self-resolved, or it may be situation–dependent. There are different degrees of impairment, from partial to total. Usually, early age of onset and total impairment indicate a difficult prognosis with a poor treatment outcome. Conversely, a history of prior adequate sexual function indicates a self-limited course and a favorable treatment outcome. Examples of problems with desire, arousal, and response follow.

Issues Regarding Desire
- Individuals who are dealing with stressful life situations such as loss of a relative, or employment instability, or have developed an illness of prolonged duration may be unable to clear their minds in order to desire any sexual experience. This problem is frequently transient and self-correcting within a reasonable period of time. Your physician may find that "adjustment disorders," a classification of psychological stresses used for diagnostic purposes, compound this problem.
- Feelings of anger or resentment directed toward the sexual partner can interfere with the ability to become sexually aroused. A recent or unresolved interpersonal dispute can be a primary factor in this matter.
- Occasionally, questions about who initiates sex may affect desire, due to culture-specific expectations or "rules" passed down from previous generations.

Issues Regarding Arousal
- Inhibition is often a factor with lack of arousal. Your physician will try to help you locate the specific sources of the inhibition.
- The inability to obtain and maintain a level of concentration on the sensuality and sexuality of the moment, whether from an external event or an internally produced

psychological trigger, may cause sexual arousal to wane or disappear. For example, an external event such as the ringing of a telephone, or an internal issue such as thinking about work-related matters (deadlines, interpersonal conflicts), may negatively impact arousal.

- In loss of arousal, when one attempts to try harder, he or she potentially becomes detached from the ability to respond to sexual stimuli. Typically, this process might begin after one or two failed experiences, regardless of external events or stresses, and then becomes an internally and negatively reinforcing cycle.

Issues Regarding Response
- Self-perceived issues concerning performance may make the ability to feel sexual become secondary to the primary frustration of being organically dysfunctional. Performance anxiety takes over and disables the ability to focus on sexual stimuli to generate a response.
- Comparisons to previous experiences may make the person worry about current sexual interactions, evaluate the intensity of one against another, and become preoccupied with making each new experience better than the preceding one.

Additionally, feelings of depression, anxiety, guilt, shame, frustration, or anger also contribute to problems of sexual desire and arousal. The extent to which such feelings affect health is measurable. The Test of Variables of Attention (TOVA) detects an individual's levels of anxiety, attention deficit, and potential for depression; its results illuminate sexual problems of desire and arousal.

In general, competent and satisfactory sexual function is considered to be associated with a healthy and adaptive personality development. Therefore, personality structure issues, accompanied by maladaptive personality traits or psychopathology, may affect sexual function. Personality profiles provide insight into characteristics of behavior and how personality affects the individual's daily approach to life, including their outlook concerning sexual encounters. We utilize a computerized Millon Clinical Multiaxial Inventory (MCMI) to determine an individual's negative characteristics, in addition to the Myers-Briggs Type Indicator (MBTI) to evaluate a person's best traits. By correlating these two testing profiles, we define a patient's personality disorders and recommend a set of exercises for behavior modification to assist in restoring a healthy personality, and to establish skills in interpersonal relations. Professional psychological counseling also may be appropriate.

Some physicians choose to administer a full neuropsychological (NP) examination that measures perception, memory, intellect, motor or tactile response, and verbal or speech ability, in addition to the TOVA and Myers-Briggs and Millon personality profiles. However, given our record with the approach outlined in Table 3, we have not found this to be a productive use of resources. We utilize only those psychological assessments that we believe will directly assist us in resolving the patient's particular issues.

The nocturnal penile tumescence study (NPT) diagnoses impotence of psychogenic origin. NPT monitors erectile function during REM, the deepest state of sleep. This technique presumes that psychological factors such as stress, emotion, and attitudes present in wakefulness are inactive in deep sleep. Organic deficits, however, would persist during sleep, and they would inhibit the number and duration of erectile episodes in sleep. Again, we have found little usefulness for NPT.

PHYSICAL AND PSYCHOLOGICAL HEALING: CRANIAL ELECTRICAL STIMULATION

Cranial Electrical Stimulation (CES) is a revolutionary new device, available by physician prescription only. Gentle electrical currents are transmitted to the brain via electrodes from a pocket-sized device. Intensity is controlled by the individual, and the procedure may be thought of as a "mind massage." Its design as an at-home therapy improves patient compliance. This modality has no relation to electroconvulsive therapy (ECT), infamous for its excessive voltage. CES therapy has been shown to positively improve brain health. It was initially introduced to the U.S. market for treatment of anxiety, depression, and insomnia, factors in health that contribute to suboptimal sexual function. CES has been shown to raise the level of conversion of amino acids into neurotransmitters and to increase blood levels of endorphins—both influence the ability for desire, arousal, and response in a sexual experience. CES may also restore proper brain wave balance. Repeated treatments have a cumulative effect, and many people find that CES promotes relaxation.

BIOFEEDBACK

Impotence of psychogenic nature is usually based in a disruption of the arousal process. The EEGs of men with arousal problems show an imbalance in cerebral hemispheric activity. Most clinical studies have demonstrated that normal sexual arousal involves an increase in activity of the nondominant hemisphere; this is not found in those individuals with lost libido.

Cases of "performance anxiety" result from cognitive attention deficits. For these men, it is difficult to focus on sexual stimuli without being preoccupied with their response during sex.

Biofeedback may help men boost their overall brain activity. Although this method does not compensate for any potential cerebral hemispheric imbalances, the objective of biofeedback is self-awareness of body functions and emotions in order to achieve self-control over any undesired activity, and the actual ability to control or direct a physical response. Such training enables an individual to become alert for his subtle, personal triggers or sensations which would be otherwise unnoticed; in this respect, a man properly trained in biofeedback may deliberately alter his behavior to suit the specific sexual situation with which he is confronted. Licensed biofeedback clinicians will first evaluate a subject for his weaker and stronger brainwaves and customize the biofeedback sessions to train the subject to adjust the waves to optimize the overall rhythm. The positive effects may include an overall enhanced sense of calm and wellness, plus an improved inner ability to focus and concentrate; these are all important contributors to the state of mind in which a pleasurable sexual experience occurs. To locate a licensed biofeedback clinician, see Resources.

CIRCULATORY ISSUES

OVERALL HEALTH

In both sexes, partial or complete failure to begin and maintain genital vasocongestion can be caused by inadequacies of the circulatory system. Occlusive vascular disease has the potential to diminish blood flow to the internal pudic arteries that supply genitalia with blood. This illness is more prevalent in men, frequently due to a deficiency of the pudic artery to properly execute the extensive branching off to supply sufficient blood flow to the penis.

Additionally, any type of condition that compromises the general cardiovascular system will compromise the ability of the penis to engorge for proper erectile function, such as:

- unhealthy lipid profile: total cholesterol, low high-density lipoprotein (HDL), high low-density lipoprotein (LDL), and high triglycerides (TGL);
- arteriosclerosis (buildup of plaque within the arteries, producing restricted blood flow);
- hypertension and perhaps side effects from medications used to treat high blood pressure; and
- factors involving the circulatory system—particularly smoking.

The initial signal of repeated failure to have an erection is an indicator that the penis is not receiving sufficient blood flow.

CHELATION THERAPY

Chelation is a process for the removal of toxic or noxious contents from the bloodstream; vitamins are often infused at the same time. When proceeding with chelation, make sure that the physician follows the standardized protocols established by the American Board of Chelation Therapy (see Resources).

Chelation uses an intravenous delivery system. It is administered over three hours in order to minimize any risk of adverse reactions to the contents of the chelating solution which usually contains:

- a carrier solution combined with ethylene diamine tetraacetic acid (EDTA), where EDTA dosage is based on body weight and assumption of normal kidney function;
- magnesium (chloride or sulfate) to minimize discomfort and as an added benefit as it is frequently deficient in those patients requiring chelation; and
- optional vitamins such as ascorbate (vitamin C), as an added benefit, which works in conjunction with EDTA for optimal toxic metal removal; B-complex vitamins, which, unfortunately, are often removed from the body during chelation; and patient-specific nutrients determined by prior analysis of vitamin deficiencies.

Most chelation patients require multiple sessions. Between sessions, the patient is screened for kidney function (specifically creatine levels) to refine the chelation process and determine the frequency required to achieve full benefit.

We use the EDTA challenge technique to evaluate the severity of patient exposure to toxicities. After loading the patient with chelating substances, we measure and analyze the postchallenge urine for heavy metals content. Additionally, chelation candidates are tested for nutritional deficiencies that may compound their specific toxic metal exposures. Our chelation regimen has demonstrated that, for certain patients, infusion of beneficial chelating amino acids (cysteine and glutathione, for example), and micronutrients (such as zinc and selenium), as well as vitamins (beta carotene), optimizes the standard chelation protocol. Our chelation protocol stabilizes cell membranes in arteries, slows the enzymes responsible for the progression of cardiovascular disease, stabilizes the electrical charge of blood platelets (reducing their "stickiness" and potential to cause clotting), and lowers arterial vasoconstriction by removing calcium and acting as a calcium-channel blocker.

When chelation is coupled with nutritional supplementation and lifestyle changes, the need for invasive techniques such as angioplasty or bypass surgery is potentially averted for cases of early cardiovascular disease. To locate a physician certified in the process of chelation, contact either the American College of Advancement in Medicine (ACAM) or the American Board of Chelation Therapy (ABCT) (see Resources).

PENILE HEALTH

Erectile difficulties or failures in men may be an inevitable effect of the aging process due to three uncontrollable cellular changes:

- As cellular tissues die (normal course of cellular cycle), they build up undesirable collections of connective tissue. This results in decreased penile distensibility.

- Changes occur in the type of collagen present in the intracavernous tissue (fibrous tubes forming the main body of the penis through which ejaculant is released). When men are young, it is elastic and pliable; as men age, the tissue becomes rigid and less able to generate erection. Additionally, this tissue buildup interferes with the ability for the nerves in the penis to communicate properly.

- Intracellular changes cause weaknesses that result in a decline of penile health.

In men without cardiac symptoms, an increased risk of myocardial infarction and stroke may correlate with low penile brachial index (PBI) values. This underscores the relationship between cardiovascular health and sexual function; even without conditions detrimental to the cardiovascular system, men are still vulnerable to decreased sexual performance.

The primary diagnostic techniques currently available for detection of improper penile function are:

- penile Doppler, a noninvasive ultrasound technique that detects constrictions or impediments in the blood flow to the penis. When used in conjunction with measurements of (a) penile systolic blood pressure or (b) brachial systolic blood pressure, to obtain the penile brachial index (PBI), this method becomes quite precise.
- cavernosonogram, where X rays are taken following the injection of a tracer dye; this procedure determines whether blood is leaking away from the penis, making it nearly impossible to maintain erection.
- penile pulse volume (PVR) recording, which analyzes the amplitude and volume of a waveform sent noninvasively through the penis; abnormal values indicate potential problems with blood flow.
- biopsy of cavernosal tissue, to analyze for presence of nitric oxide synthase (NOS), which is correlated with the integrity of the penile nerves. This method allows for determination of neurogenic impotence as caused by cavernous nerve damage.
- angiography, a technique which involves injection of a medium for which its flow through blood vessels is monitored to detect arterial disease.
- nocturnal penile tumescence (NPT) study.

Under development are many new procedures for the diagnosis of vascular health of the penis.

ERECTILE PRODUCTION

The Medicated Urethral System for Erection (MUSE) is a method for delivering alprostadil, a type of prostaglandin-1, via the urethral tube. It induces erection by relaxing penile smooth muscle tissue while dilating the cavernosal arteries, resulting in an engorgement of blood to the penis. MUSE inserts are effective regardless of the age of the subject or the organic cause of erectile dysfunction—including vascular disease, diabetes, surgery, or trauma. The MUSE begins working within five to ten minutes of administration, and holds for up to thirty minutes. It is not for use unless impotence is validated; used improperly, it may cause permanent penile damage. Some men experience minor pain at the entry site, but not significant enough to defer from intercourse.

Papaverine is a vasodilating substance. When a 15 to 20 percent papaverine base gel is applied to male genitalia, increased blood flow to the penis results. Minimal systemic absorption occurs, and no toxicity from the topical application is reported. Papaverine gel is compounded by specialty pharmacies; your physician will make the arrangements to acquire this product if appropriate.

Another option is to produce erections by intracavernosal (spongy tissue area of penis) injection of vasodilating substances. Reflex erections can be elicited by locally administered substances designed to dilate the penile blood vessels to cause increased blood flow to erectile tissue. We do not usually employ this technique, as MUSE inserts or papaverine gel have been successful.

HORMONES

INTRODUCTION

The body produces a variety of hormones for many biological functions. Of these hormones, testosterone, dehydroepiandrosterone, prolactin, growth hormone and insulin growth factors, and melatonin are directly relevant to sexual function. Thyroid hormones are important, too, because any imbalances may lead to pituitary or hypothalamic failure which affects production of the sex-related hormones.

It is critically important that the body maintain a homeostatic level of hormones for proper body function. The body constantly monitors its hormonal blood levels in order to produce them in the necessary amounts.

TESTOSTERONE

In men and women, testosterone is produced by the adrenal glands. Testosterone is also produced in the sexual organs: a significant amount is produced in men (testes); a small amount in premenopausal women (ovaries). For a long time, testosterone was considered to be the hormone of aggression. However, recent research actually shows that a shortage of testosterone may cause aggression, and that estrogen increases physically aggressive behaviors and aggressive impulses. Indeed, there are many clinical benefits for testosterone replacement therapy in men (see Table 4). See Bibliography for published scientific research.

Table 4.
Potential Benefits of Natural Testosterone Therapy for Men

- Sex drive/potency increase
- Cardiovascular system improvement
- Circulatory system improvement
- Muscular strength improvement
- Skeletal system improvement
- Cholesterol profile improvement; potential reduction in risk of coronary heart disease
- Improved self-perceived wellness
- Leaner body mass
- Minimization of bone loss
- Stabilization of blood sugar
- Hematological improvement
- For peripheral vascular disease
- For muscle cramps
- For liver function
- For Alzheimer's disease, dementia
- For pregangrene condition

EXERCISE TO RAISE TESTOSTERONE LEVELS

The most natural way to increase serum testosterone is through physical training, which also benefits overall physical health. Develop an appropriate exercise regimen on the advice of your physician. When exercise is conducted properly, heart volume rises, oxygen is used efficiently, and testosterone production is increased. Six months of physical training may increase the volume of the red cells in the blood, as well as the testosterone level, as much as 20 percent. Men in fit physical condition can raise their testosterone level up to 40 percent, whereas those lesser trained can raise it approximately 15 percent.

REPLACEMENT WITH NATURAL FORMS OF TESTOSTERONE

Synthetically produced testosterone was initially introduced to the market in pill form—methyl testosterone. It is no longer prescribed because it is a form of testosterone that has been linked to liver cancer. Fortunately, a few different forms of testosterone supplements are available at the present time. We find that the best form is natural testosterone—testosterone undecanoate—produced from plant sources. The pill or capsule version, taken orally, is absorbed in the gastrointestinal system and goes from the blood stream to the liver, being neutralized before it serves a beneficial use. As a result, the blood level of testosterone cannot be raised using oral administration for some men.

Injections of testosterone are essentially natural in that they are identical to human testosterone. Administered intramuscularly every two to four weeks, there are negative aspects to this form of supplementation as well: the needle injection can be uncomfortable, and the level of circulating testosterone in the blood declines between injections. As the testosterone level falls, some men may experience anxiety, fatigue, feelings of anger or depression, and a decline in sexual activity.

Because of the difficulties some patients have with testosterone injections, attempts made to develop alternative methods to deliver testosterone yielded sublingual administration as well as slow-release microcapsules implanted just under the skin.

The next generation of testosterone delivery to be established was a safe, convenient, self-applied, self-adhesive patch from which the hormone is delivered into the body with a constancy over a twenty-four-hour period. The initial patch product, available since the early 1980s, was applied to the scrotum, where the skin is rapidly permeable. However, there were difficulties with scrotal patch testosterone: the patch could fall off if the individual were sweating excessively or when the scrotal skin contracted (a normal occurrence). Medically, the potential for the adverse effect of elevated dihydrotestosterone (DHT) caused by overactivity of an enzyme released by the scrotum (possibly in response to the patch) was of concern; high DHT levels had been linked to increased potential for prostate cancer.

We now prescribe the newest testosterone patch if we find testosterone deficiencies. A testosterone transdermal system may be applied to the midriff area, thighs, and outer arms—multiple locations are used on a rotating basis to minimize the minor side effect of skin irritation. This product does not create excess scrotal DHT production similar to the scrotal patch. Not only does the transdermal product have a duration of twenty-four hours, it also delivers testosterone in a manner that simulates normal testosterone fluctuation. Because it is applied at bedtime, the testosterone in this system gradually rises throughout the morning, peaking at midday, then begins a gentle decline until evening, when a fresh patch is applied. The testosterone transdermal system has revolutionized testosterone supplementation options, as it eliminates the mood swings associated with injection therapy, and remains securely attached despite active exercise. Most patients report revitalization in both overall and sexual health within three weeks of the first patch usage. This product, however, is not indicated for (1) men with breast cancer; (2) men with suspected or actual prostate cancer; or (3) women.

Replacement using naturally-based testosterone therapy is considered to be very safe and effective when properly supervised. Testosterone supplementation should be given by an experienced doctor, since it can sometimes cause an enlarged prostate and may provoke prostate cancer growth. To combat the potential for prostate enlargement, use saw palmetto extract (an herbal derivative) in combination with zinc. Testosterone patients should have a regular prostate exam, as well as special blood work for prostate cancer named PSA (prostate specific antigen) on a regular schedule deemed appropriate for the intensity of the individual's testosterone therapy. Minor incidences of priapism (persistent erection) have been noted in clinical studies.

DEHYDROEPIANDROSTERONE (DHEA)

DHEA is a ubiquitous steroid-based hormone, and its presence throughout the body outmeasures others in its class. DHEA is converted to DHEA-S (dehydroepiandrosterone sulfate)—its active form, where it proceeds to various sites in the body. Of particular interest is the function of DHEA as a mild androgen. When it is used in conjunction with testosterone therapy, it acts similarly to corticosteroids but with a reduction in the negative side effects that are produced by administration of testosterone alone. Two weeks of DHEA replacement in healthy men and women between the ages of forty and seventy resulted in DHEA and DHEA-S levels found in young adults, with the increases persisting throughout the study period. Additionally, the rise in DHEA levels correlated with improvement of overall physical and psychological wellness, without side effects from the supplementation.

Determination of DHEA levels are sometimes a more accurate indicator of impotence than testosterone testing. Where DHEA-S measurements are elevated, hyperprolactinemia is indicated. If DHEA-S levels are elevated yet testosterone is within normal range, an excess production of androgens, possibly due to malfunctions in the adrenal glands, is the cause.

DHEA REPLACEMENT

Studies at our facility have shown that decreased levels of DHEA correlate with sexual dysfunction, premature aging, and inability to handle stress. From blood testing, we have determined that DHEA levels begin to decline at approximately the age of thirty. Replacement dosages are age-based.

The benefits of DHEA supplementation usually outweigh any ill effects it may cause. Supplementation potentially elevates dihydroxytestosterone (DHT) levels. DHT, a potent androgen that does not participate in pertinent male biosynthesis reactions, may be indicated in prostate illness. By monitoring DHT, DHEA, DHEA-S, and cortisol levels, and prescribing antidotal supplements, DHEA supplementation may be safely continued. If prostate disease is suspected conduct DHEA supplementation carefully: the ultimate product of DHEA is testosterone, which may exacerbate prostate troubles because prostate cancer is a hormonally-based illness. Additionally, DHEA supplementation may produce imbalances in thyroid hormones and immune-system cells.

PROLACTIN

Prolactin is important in maintaining a functional pituitary; normal pituitary function is critical to homeostatic hormone levels throughout the body.

Elevated DHEA levels may indicate hyperprolactinemia, which interferes with the transport of dopamine to the pituitary. Common characteristics of hyperprolactinemia include decreased libido, suppression of sexual interest, and possible infertility. Hyperprolactinemia may lead to increased incidences of headaches, as well as the onset of diabetes insipidus [the pituitary fails to produce antidiuretic hormone (ADH)]—with symptoms of enormous volumes of urine and excessive thirst. Left untreated, this condition may cause irreversible loss of vision, because of pressure exerted by the enlarged pituitary gland on the optic nerve. Prolactin-secreting microadenomas may be formed—frequently benign neoplasms affecting the pituitary gland. In men, the growth may decrease sexual interest by physically prohibiting the pituitary's ability to continue to signal the testes to produce testosterone.

Unfortunately, the majority of the medical community recommends surgical correction of prolactin-secreting microadenomas; often accompanying surgery is administration of bromocriptine to continue the inhibition of prolactin. Radiation to reduce the size of the growth is often used. At our practice, we monitor the neoplasms for their actual affect on the patient's health: many of these neoplasms may be redefined as "pituitary incidental-omas"—meaning that they are afflictions which are not medically significant. When the growths begin to interfere with overall or sexual health, treatment with tyrosine, an amino acid, or dopamine D2-agonists are nonsurgical alternatives. The appropriateness of such treatment course varies among individual patients.

GROWTH HORMONE

Growth hormone, or somatotropin, is secreted by the pituitary gland and causes the release of somatomedins from the liver. Growth hormone causes the growth of muscle and bone and releases energy from the breakdown of fat.

Novel studies have posited strong correlations that growth hormone may affect the brain's abilities in cognition, emotion, and mood, and boost cellular metabolism, leading to increased energy: such general effects have a decisive impact upon the individual's sexual interest and ability to respond. Growth hormone has also been associated with increased libido, pleasure in response, and potential for multiple orgasms.

Testing for growth hormone is useful in the diagnosis of hypothalamic disorders or hypopituitarism. Currently, the most reliable method is by stimulatory testing, which can clearly discern an underactive thyroid.

GROWTH HORMONE REPLACEMENT

Deficiency of somatotrophin must first be verified prior to initiation of growth hormone therapy. Additionally, since some studies indicate that growth hormone replacement may worsen the levels of thyroid hormone production, it is prudent to conduct thyroid testing to evaluate for hypothyroidism.

Growth hormone therapy is delivered using a synthetic preparation. Its replacement is frequently combined with that of other hormones, to achieve a synergistic result. Growth hormone therapy carries a minimal risk of the development of diabetes mellitus during the course of treatment; when properly monitored, prolonged treatment will not have this result.

INSULIN GROWTH FACTORS (IGFs)

IGFs are a set of the body's "superhormones"—they have the ability to alter the levels of other, subservient hormones. In the case of IGFs, they affect growth hormone levels. IGF measurement is useful to monitor the progress of growth hormone therapy.

Insulin-like growth factors (IGF-1,-3, and -C), are secreted by the pituitary via stimulation from growth hormone. IGFs are produced in the liver, influencing the growth of bone and muscle, as well as the metabolism of minerals, carbohydrates, and fats. When IGF levels are high, the levels of sex hormone–binding globulin (SHBG) are low. Circulating amounts of free (unbound) testosterone levels correspond to IGF levels. We use the SHBG test as a marker for levels of testosterone: if SHBG is low, so is testosterone.

The importance of the IGF class on age-related diseases requires further examination: there are indications that low concentrations of IGF-1 correlate with nonfunctioning pituitary tumors. Typical IGF levels found in men are 100–200 ng/mL; the goal of supplementation is to raise the values to 500 ng/mL.

MELATONIN

Melatonin is produced at the pineal gland, which is a light-sensitive organ that contains pigment cells, similar to those of the eyes. Because the pineal gland produces its hormone during periods of darkness, secretions of melatonin are most pronounced during sleep. Melatonin is produced from tryptophan, an amino acid, and serotonin, a neurotransmitter derived from tryptophan.

With regard to sexual activity, melatonin is important because the pineal gland is capable of detecting declines in gonadal hormones. It is speculated that melatonin makes sex more pleasurable by stimulating the desire for sex, encouraging intimacy, and heightening the effect of endorphins (a product of the pituitary gland which regulates mood) during sex.

Melatonin is not readily tested by blood specimen because of variable factors such as time of day that the specimen is drawn and quantity or quality of sleep. Thus, alertness to signals from the body is the method in which low melatonin levels are mostly detected; in essence, the irregularity of melatonin may be self-diagnosed. Low levels of melatonin predict sleep disorders—specifically, irregular patterns. As a secondary effect, the individual may become irritable and easily agitated; this certainly impacts the chances for sexual experiences to occur.

MELATONIN REPLACEMENT

Intake of melatonin may be relevant in boosting sexual function. However, the process of replenishment is slow, as the melatonin first proceeds to neurological, immunological, and sleep-generating systems, and then to its final action in enhancing sexual status. Melatonin secretion may be boosted using testosterone injections. Testosterone has a renormalizing effect on the activity pattern associated with melatonin production.

BENEFICIAL OPTIONS THAT MAY HELP IN REGAINING SEXUAL VITALITY

NUTRITIONAL OPTIONS

The use of dietary supplements (vitamins, minerals, and herbs) to boost ailing libido and sexual function is becoming commonplace. However, it is critical for a physician to first determine your blood levels of vitamins, trace elements (minute quantities of beneficial minerals), amino acids, and essential fatty acids (cellular energy source). Screening for negative blood content such as exposure to toxic products or heavy metals may also be important (see Environmental Issues). By reviewing these test results in light of any preexisting medical conditions, your physician is prepared to implement a properly constructed nutritional supplementation program for your needs.

Keep in mind that any supplementation program will require a period of adjustment of the individual's body to the added nutrients—after all, the concentrated nutrient, though beneficial, may be novel to the body. Alterations in dosage are often appropriate in order to achieve the ideal combination. After the adjustment phase, and once the proper dosages are determined, the body is able to expedite its process of recovery.

Vitamins that are necessary for proper blood circulation, such as niacin (a form of vitamin B3) and vitamin E, are valid candidates to improve sexual function.

Amino acids, a group of twenty-nine molecular "building blocks" used throughout the body to manufacture proteins, are utilized for a wide array of body functions, most importantly: to produce neurotransmitters; to manufacture cellular fuel; to stabilize blood sugar, blood pressure, and mood; and for responses such as detoxification, immunity, or healing. Abnormalities for which correction may exert positive effects include:

- improvement in endocrine function
- increased energy and stamina
- reduced aggression
- improved condition of cardiovascular system
- pain relief, including arthritis
- antidepressant effects

Recent research has shown that the level of arginine, a precursor to nitric oxide synthase (NOS), may be important to sexual health. Carnitine may combat cardiovascular illness by decreasing high TGL levels while increasing HDLs. Tyrosine may increase sex drive by stimulating adrenal hormone production and increasing energy levels.

Prostaglandin E1 (10–40 mcg) may also be appropriate in assisting libido. The prostaglandin class is a group of three types of internally produced lipids, important for their effect as hormones performing at various sites upon delivery. These hormones differ from the endocrine version in that they are produced in cells throughout the body for local secretion and immediate action. Prostaglandins—perhaps in their ubiquitous presence within the body—have been observed to affect all major functions of the body, sexual performance being no exception. Prostaglandins are the active component in MUSE inserts. The precursors to prostaglandins are essential fatty acids, EFAs. As supplied in supplement form (which is derived from fish oils), EFAs perform dual-duty in the body: it has been indicated that they aid in cardiovascular issues as well as assist in transmission of nerve impulses, specifically within the brain. It is noteworthy that direct prostaglandin therapy may cause burning sensations; because EFA supplementation raises prostaglandin E1 levels, it is prudent to utilize the former to assist in remedying sexual difficulties.

There is a potential correlation between nutritional supplements utilized for infertility to assist in overall sexual health. A regimen possibly including vitamin C (up to 3 g daily), B-complex, antioxidants, EFAs, vitamin E, magnesium, and extra doses of zinc (a main component in semen) has been shown to benefit fertility. This postulation is derived from the fact that supplements utilized to produce increases in quality and quantity of sperm and semen—with the goal of improved fertility—may also benefit men experiencing difficulty in resolution.

LIFESTYLE CHANGES

Regular aerobic exercise (under your physician's approval) is essential for maintaining proper cardiovascular and circulatory conditions. Without proper blood circulation, sexual function is compromised.

Basic good health recommendations for diet include (verify with your physician):

- protein (meat)—beneficial for the body in that it is a major source for amino acids—fish and chicken are ideal; nuts, eggs, dairy products are alternative protein sources
- whole-grain products
- vegetables and fruit

- polyunsaturated or monosaturated oils
- spring and mineral waters

Reduce or avoid sugar, sugar substitutes, and alcohol, as well as additives, fillers, and preservatives. Additionally, foods high in zinc (such as oysters), thyroid-stimulating foods (such as those containing iodine), and items containing cortisone-like substances (such as the herb sarsaparilla) may assist sexual drive by boosting hormone production. Certainly, an increased quantity of such foods will have to be made a part of a basic, well-balanced diet. Interestingly, some foods will reduce sexual function; these include thyroid-inhibitors (cabbage family), purely vegan diets, and excesses of sugar and chocolate. (Verify the impact of any of these suggestions as they may pertain to your specific health conditions with your physician prior to use.)

COUNSELING WITH A LICENSED SEX THERAPIST OR COUPLES COUNSELOR

It is important for couples to seek professional assistance to deal with their own emotions concerning suboptimal sexual performance as well as to understand those of their partner. Left unaddressed, the initial issue may become compounded by other factors and jeopardize the couple's relationship. Issues over which one has little control—such as illnesses like diabetes mellitus, or advanced cardiovascular or circulatory disease—can precipitate the need for a third-party with which a couple can mitigate their emotions. There are several organizations from which couples may obtain referrals to qualified therapists (see Resources).

ABSTINENCE

Abstinence has been studied in reference to issues of fertility; determination of sperm quality and motility all have been evaluated. This guide does not address the nuances of infertility treatment. However, a review of the literature concerning the usage of abstinence to enhance fertility does yield some insight for the issue of increasing sexual response.

A period of sexual abstinence between two to five days

increases the number of sperm contained in ejaculated semen; interestingly, refraining from sexual activity for a period beyond seven days generally produces decreased sperm count.

For men not concerned with reproduction, abstinence may shorten the time needed to achieve erection, reduce the need for physical stimulation of the penis by the partner, assist in maintenance of the erection through completion of sexual activity, and increase the man's sense of satisfaction. Such abstinence for two to five days may provide some improvement in sexual performance. It is a method which can be conducted without special medical advice (unless contraindicated by an illness or not recommended by your physician).

MASTURBATION

Masturbation is medically valid but is somewhat of a social taboo. It is a method enabling retention of normal penile functions. Regular sexual activity of any kind, either via masturbation or with a partner, is a necessary and normal component of male sexual fitness. Without it, self confidence may wane and with it, so may sexual freedom.

ADDITIONAL IMPORTANT MEDICAL ISSUES FOR SEXUAL FITNESS

PROSTATE HEALTH

The health of the prostate is an important indicator of a variety of potential problems: sexual, urological, and cancer risk. Any symptoms concerning urination, such as difficulty with the process (starting or ceasing flow), weak and irregular flow, or increased frequency require an immediate physical exam and assessment. Additional signs of potential prostate illness are pains in the pelvic region, back, or upper thighs.

The Prostate Specific Antigen (PSA) test is the most accurate detector for adenocarcinomas of the prostate. Where PSA levels are elevated, it indicates a sign of either benign or malignant cancer. Regularly scheduled screenings, preferably conducted in conjunction with a digital rectal examination, may increase an individual's awareness of the significance of the prostate in its function on a sexual and nonsexual level.

It has been postulated that melatonin may be valuable as an adjunct to conventional treatment for enlarged prostate or benign prostate hypertrophy, as it may mimic the mechanism of prescription medications used for these conditions.

NEUROPATHIES

Neuropathies are disorders which affect the nervous system, causing debilitated function of sensory and motor capacities. These illnesses are typically associated with diabetics and with alcohol and drug abusers. The unfortunate difficulty with such men is that they are unable to detect the problem because of neural damage. Treatment with vitamin B12 injections, electrical stimulation, and methods to improve the neurological system may help; however, in general the prognosis is fair-to-poor because of a lack of early intervention.

OBESITY

Obesity poses multiple health issues. Obesity correlates to unhealthy hormone levels: obese men aged twenty to seventy possess low serum testosterone level plus excess insulin and glucose values. Obese men often possess higher diastolic blood pressure readings and increased LDLs, factors that negatively affect overall health. Obesity also may cause muscles in the midriff and upper thigh areas to atrophy, possibly creating issues for performance in sex. Obese men are jeopardizing their sexual function as well as increasing their chances for coronary heart disease and potential onset of diabetes.

After placing abdominally obese middle-aged men on transdermal testosterone, adipose tissue triglycerides may decrease while the turnover of lipids in the abdominal adipose tissue region may increase. Additional effects potentially include notable decreases in visceral fat, plasma cholesterol and triglycerides, (fasting) glucose, and diastolic blood pressure. Testosterone may be beneficial for obese men to restore cardiovascular health, deter against diabetes onset, and regain sexual wellness. Careful physician supervision of testosterone treatment for any man, obese or not, is crucial to detect changes in prostate health, PSA results, or urological disorders.

In obese men with higher values of visceral fat (versus subcutaneous or total fat) and elevated systolic blood pressure and triglycerides, low concentrations of IGF-1 may be found. This may indicate that low IGF-1 correlates to deficient or depressed growth hormone production. Typical IGF levels found in men are 100–200 ng/mL; the goal of supplementation is to raise the values to 500 ng/mL.

To correct weakened midriff and thigh muscles, consult your physician and perhaps a physical therapist and fitness instructor to devise a program of anaerobic weightlifting and exercise which will assist in restoring proper muscular function.

DIABETES MELLITUS

The incident that precipitates the onset of diabetes mellitus may be neurogenic, vascular, or due to an alteration in muscular function. In male patients with diabetes mellitus, it is estimated that within five years of onset of illness the vast majority will experience some type of sexual dysfunction. Regardless of the duration of the illness, men over the age of forty with diabetes mellitus will have a higher incidence of erectile failure. In men aged twenty to fifty with diabetes mellitus, a majority report sexual dysfunction. It is suspected that insulin deficiencies cause a rise in prolactin and dehydroepiandrosterone (DHT) levels, potentially leading to inhibition of testosterone secretion. Some men with diabetes mellitus may also experience disorders with spermatogenesis, partially due to hypotrophy (reduction in structure) of the testes.

Cases of diabetes mellitus of an organic origin frequently correlate to diminished serum-free testosterone levels; this is not the case for diabetic men whose cases are psychogenic in nature. Treatment solely with glucose-monitoring usually will not improve the sexual performance of the organic-based diabetic group. In diabetic men with no evidence of penile vascular disease, testosterone therapy may assist in erectile activity as well as improve self-perceived sexual performance.

At our practice, we have found that diabetics who begin growth hormone therapy have a greater opportunity for recovery of sexual function than diabetics who do not.

PRESCRIPTION AND OVER-THE-COUNTER MEDICATIONS

In today's world, too many people are taking multiple medications for prolonged periods of time. It is well established that medications for all classes of hypertensive drugs, antidepressants, antimania, antipsychotics, antianxiety, antifungals, and anticoagulants all potentially impair sexual desire and performance. To avoid potential overmedication, alert your physician to all over-the-counter medications you take, and verify that all prescription medications are listed in your medical file.

If a prescribed pharmaceutical is suspected of interfering with sexual desire, your physician should recommend you temporarily discontinue it in order to make a diagnostic evaluation. "Drug holidays" must be closely supervised by your physician. The side effects of prescriptions may be reversed by reduction of the dosage, or ideally, discontinuation of the medication. Prescription medications frequently have specific negative side effects relating to sexual function, for example, some may cause priapism (chronic erection) or sexual hypofunction (loss of drive).

ALCOHOL AND DRUG ABUSE

Alcohol or other substance abuse can cause decreased sexual desire. In younger men, illicit drugs are the most common causes of organic impotence. Excesses of alcohol and usage of any illicit drug may cause permanent physical and psychological impairments. If loss of sexual drive is secondary to alcohol or substance abuse, it is imperative to find the exact offenders by means of laboratory screening. Treatment should aim to control, and ultimately cease, the abuse. Long-term alcohol or substance abuse can cause irreversible damage to the liver. Overall health, and sexual health as well, will then decline sharply.

Professional counseling is an invaluable tool for alcoholics or substance abusers. For a list of organizations offering referrals to appropriate counselors, see Resources. Additionally, the complete emotional support of family members—partners, children, and extended family—plus close friends, is essential because they can form a responsive, understanding network with whom the individual may confront their issues.

DYSFUNCTIONS OF OTHER ORIGINS

Individuals with coronary artery diseases, especially post-myocardial patients, have specific issues caused by their illness that affect sexual function. The management of such issues is closely related to proper postinfarction rehabilitation. Loss of desire may be secondary to psychological factors such as stress, anger, and fear, and can further complicate interpersonal problems. Such difficulties are ameliorated by counseling. A rare problem that some postoperative patients may experience is unwarranted or unwanted erections. Anti-androgen or antifungal medications may be administered to minimize or prevent this condition. Your physician will determine proper treatment.

Men with spinal cord injury (SCI) suffer from difficulties with sexual function, primarily due to inadequate or poorly sustained erections. The recovery to normalized sexual function is more difficult for men with SCI who are experiencing neurogenic-based dysfunction. Many of these men are young when injured, so impotence may have existed for a long time. Other skeletal problems such as lumbar disk pain and chronic prostatitis may also contribute to sexual dysfunction.

Nitroglycerin plasters of papaverine applied to the penis have been successful in producing erections in men with SCI. However, recent research shows that papaverine injection is more likely to produce erections, and is necessary if men require more papaverine than that provided in the plasters. Priapism is a potential side effect with the intracavernous option. Intracavernous injection of prostaglandin E1 for SCI men may produce functional erection, without systemic side effects.

Injury to the cavernous nerve (which leads from the torso to the penis) and associated genital nerves may happen during surgery to remove pelvic tumors or during urological procedures for prostate cancer, bladder cancer, or colorectal surgery. The nerve damage may cause failures in neurotransmission signals that normally trigger penile arousal and response. Advances in surgical methods minimize the risk, but some postoperative dysfunction may occur due to pre-existing malfunctions in the cavernous arteries (those vessels which fill with blood to cause penile rigidity).

FREE RADICAL DAMAGE

Free radicals are extremely reactive atoms that readily bond. For a molecule to be stable, all of its atoms must have all of its electrons (negatively charged ions) paired with positrons (positively charged ions) in all orbits. Free radicals are aggressive in their ability to bond because they have unpaired electrons—either due to an odd number of electrons or to a single unpaired electron in a readily bonding location (the outermost orbit around the atom).

Free radicals are able to convert stable, nonradical compounds by forcibly knocking into them, causing the latter to lose or gain an electron from the free radical: by gaining the electron, the molecule is converted into free-radical form; by losing the electron, it is readily able to pair with the initiating free radical. From that point, a chain reaction occurs as concurrent side-reactions generate additional free radical compounds.

Free radicals contribute to aging by weakening the brain tissue. Brain tissue is specifically vulnerable because free radicals "feast" on lipids (fat molecules). Lipids are found in great quantity in the brain. They are a main component of neurons (messenger cells that carry electrical impulses throughout the nervous system), and the brain contains the highest concentration of neurons. Over time—as we age—the continual and unchecked free radical destruction of brain neurons will disable the brain's ability to control and signal the endocrine, cardiovascular, circulatory, muscular, skeletal, and immunological systems properly.

There are three primary methods by which free radical damage is halted. They include:

- Nutritional control. At this time, the best remedy is oral intake of antioxidant supplements such as beta-carotene, vitamin C, and vitamin E. As a free radical chain reaction proliferates, its reactivity lessens each time. The purpose of an antioxidant is to use it to bond to a weak free radical and disable it from continuing its cycle. B-complex vitamins are also important. Also useful are trace elements such as magnesium which is frequently displaced by toxic metals, and selenium and zinc, which should also be supplemented.
- The bonding of some free radicals with each other to form a stable molecule, thus terminating two atoms.
- The automatic termination of certain free radical cycles by certain enzymatic pathways.

ENVIRONMENTAL ISSUES

TOXIC EXPOSURES

In today's world, it is difficult to find any location in the U.S. totally absent of toxins. The toxic waste dumping at Love Canal in New York State and the radioactive leakage at

Three Mile Island Nuclear Plant in Pennsylvania are glaring, frightening images of blatant toxic exposures. However, factories, gas-powered vehicles, and chemicals used to clean the home or workplace, or present in other products such as paint, plastics, upholstery, and personal items such as beauty products not only pollute our environment but our bodies as well. Vulnerabilities to the items in Table 5 contribute to decline in overall, as well as sexual, health.

Table 5.
Toxic Heavy Metals Exposures

Metal	Exposure
Aluminum, lead, cadmium, arsenic, copper, mercury	Inhaled as fumes or ingested from paints, chemicals, gasoline. Aluminum leaches from canned foods; cadmium is present in cigarettes; mercury has been a component in dental amalgams
Organic chemicals	Solvents from paints, paint thinner, nail polish/remover; industrial-strength cleaners; dry cleaning fumes; carpet, furniture, and car interior outgassing
Fungicides, insecticides, herbicides, pesticides	Inhaled during use on plants or ingested with food
Preservatives and dyes	Ingested with food

Prevention of exposure through avoidance is the optimal approach. The adverse effects of toxic metals are still being explored, but we know that elevated levels of toxic metals in the bloodstream reduce its capacity to carry beneficial minerals. Prepare your food properly: (1) make food selections carefully, (2) wash food thoroughly before preparing or eating it, (3) do not prepare recipes containing acidic ingredients (such as tomatoes, citrus, or vinegars) in aluminum cookware because the aluminum may be deposited into the food, and (4) reduce your consumption of foods sold in cans.

CHELATION THERAPY

Chelation may help to reverse the "rusting out" caused by toxic metals. Conditions involving memory loss, depression, psychosis, degenerative systemic diseases, elevated blood pressure, depression, or rheumatoid arthritis—when symptomatic of toxic exposures—may be improved. The extent and speed of recovery from these illnesses via chelation varies with the individual patient. The primary side effects observed have been fatigue and diuretic effects.

OTHER APPROACHES

MEDICATION TO CREATE ERECTIONS

Yohimbine hydrochloride, when orally administered, may alter sympathetic nerve impulses and result in an increased blood flow to the genitals. This medication has been reported to improve sexual function in about 50 percent of men with either organic or psychogenic impotence. Sometimes, three weeks are required in order for the increase in genital blood circulation to occur. The occasional side effects include nausea, dizziness, or nervousness; possible hypertension may occur in some patients. Yohimbine is contraindicated for persons with kidney disease, and not recommended for those with liver disease.

Despite the possible side effects, yohimbine continues to be utilized because of its efficacy in correcting sexual dysfunction. A trial on patients with psychogenic impotence found that 5.4 mg of yohimbine three times per day improves sexual function in 62 percent (18 of 29 people), compared to only 16 percent (3 of 19 people) in the control group. Even among those with medical disorders, as many as 43 percent will still improve with yohimbine at 5.4 mg three times a day; some men may require eight tablets daily.

Furthermore, yohimbine can correct sexual function that has been inhibited by antidepressant medication. Men using yohimbine must be monitored for potential hypertension.

MEDICATION TO TREAT PREMATURE EJACULATION

Sexual dysfunction that has been traced to a psychogenic origin, specifically anxiety, may be alleviated by antidepressants (paroxetine hydrochloride) or anti-obsessional medication (clomipramine hydrochloride). These medications may assist men afflicted with anxiety-based premature ejaculation.

SURGERY

When a disease process has caused permanent impairment of neurological, vascular, or other anatomical functioning in males, a surgical option may be appropriate. Currently, there are two types of penile prosthetic devices which allow impotent men to engage in intercourse. The Small/Keron prosthesis is a set of semirigid rods that are placed in the penis, allowing the man to create a permanent and modest erection. The second type of prosthesis is also completely implanted; this device operates by inflation of a hydraulic cylinder to permit stiffening of the penis, and deflation to control its return to flaccidity.

The most common indication for implantation of penile prosthetic devices has been in impotent diabetics who are otherwise healthy; other reasons are in cases of irreversible arteriosclerosis damage or spinal cord injury. Additionally, this method of treatment is also effective for men with neurogenic dysfunction versus those with vascular or other illnesses.

Counseling of the patient and his spouse or partner is an essential element of a rehabilitative program before and after surgery.

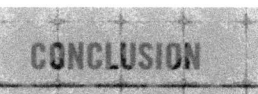
CONCLUSION

There are four categories of body functions to which ailing sexual fitness may most often be attributed:

- Brain state
- Circulatory state
- Endocrine state
- Neurological state of penis

Each of these functions is greatly affected by one's nutritional state.

To compound the issue of lost libido, some medical conditions adversely affect sex drive and performance. Many cases respond to a combination of treatments to correct brain physical and psychological factors, enhance venous and arterial circulation, and replace hormone deficits; sometimes erectile-producing agents are appropriate.

If medications are indicated, they should be prescribed at the lowest possible dosage for the shortest period of time. Long-term dependence on pharmaceuticals does not provide overall health benefits. It is imperative that treatment does not generate secondary illnesses or contribute to a decline in your emotional wellness.

In the future, we expect that more physicians will adopt multimodal techniques to evaluate and treat illnesses. Through a combination of brain mapping, psychological evaluations, blood tests, and noninvasive ultrasound techniques, our practice is able to accurately and promptly identify factors affecting sexual wellness. An integrative treatment approach is the most effective way that physicians can help their patients. Illness is most speedily tackled by using a variety of techniques. No man should be expected to consider his sexual drive and function to be permanently lost.

Androgen: a set of hormones that causes the secondary sex characteristics such as facial hair, deepening of voice, increase in muscle bulk.

Cowper's glands (2): excretory ducts passing into the urethra; they diminish in size with advancing age.

Hormone: functions include regulating the body's metabolic rate, growth, and sexual development and function. Hormones are secreted by glands in the brain and throughout the torso; sex-related hormones are produced in the testes (in men) and ovaries (in women). All hormones are released directly into the bloodstream for rapid transport to the target organs and tissues.

Neurotransmitter: messenger in the nervous system that carries signals between an initiating site and target location.

Penis: delivers ejaculant fluid (mixture of sperm and seminal fluid).

Prostate gland: produces 30 percent of the seminal fluid. Approximately the size of a walnut. The prostate is next to the bladder and urethra; its ducts open into the urethra.

Scrotum: a sac which houses the two testes. It is composed of muscle tissue.

Seminal vesicles (2): produce 70 percent of the seminal fluid.

Testes (2): each testicle is approximately the size of an apricot. This is the site at which sperm mature and are held until released with the seminal fluid as ejaculant.

Vas deferens: the excretory duct of the testes.

FURTHER READING

Braverman, E., M.D. *PATH Wellness Manual.* Princeton, N.J.: Publications for Achieving Total Health, 1995. [Available exclusively from PATH Medical. Call (212) 213-6155 for ordering information.]

Braverman, E., M.D., Carl Pfeiffer, M.D., Ken Blum, M.D., and Richard Smayda, D.O. *The Healing Nutrients Within,* 2d. ed. Los Angeles: Keats Publishing, 1997.

Casdorph, Richard, M.D., Ph.D., and Morton Walker, DPM. *Toxic Metal Syndrome.* Garden City Park, N.Y.: Avery Publishing Group, 1995.

Klatz, Ronald, and Carol Kahn. *Grow Young with HGH.* New York: HarperCollins Publishers, Inc., 1997.

Moller, J. *Cholesterol.* New York: Springer-Verlag, 1987.

Montague, Droko, M.D. *Disorders of Male Sexual Function.* Chicago: Year-Book Medical Publishers, Inc., 1988.

Pfeiffer, Carl, M.D. *Zinc and Other Micronutrients.* Los Angeles: Keats Publishing, 1978.

Pierpaoli, Walter, M.D., and William Regelson, MD. *The Melatonin Miracle.* New York: Simon & Schuster, 1995.

Rosen, Raymond C., and J. Gayle Beck. *Patterns of Sexual Arousal: Psychophysiological Processes and Clinical Applications.* New York: The Guilford Press, 1988.

Shealy, C. Norman, M.D., Ph.D. *DHEA: The Youth and Health Hormone.* Los Angeles: Keats Publishing, 1996.

THE PLACE FOR ACHIEVING TOTAL HEALTH—PATH MEDICAL

The PATH approach to disease operates on a multimodal basis for diagnosis and treatment; it is unique in that it combines state-of-the-art computerized technology to identify early stages of illness. The objective is to determine the role of brain chemical and psychological health on illness. If the brain fails to function optimally, it does not signal parts of the body to perform at their full potential. PATH Medical is a full-service family health care center that is dedicated to mind/body medicine. To find out more, call our office in New York City [(212) 213-6155] or visit our Web site at http://www.pathmed.com.

CHELATION

To locate certified physicians following American Board of Chelation Therapy Protocol, contact:

American Board of Chelation Therapy (ABCT)
Chicago, IL 60610; (312) 787-2228

American College of Advancement of Medicine (ACAM)
Laguna Hills, CA; (714) 586-7666

BIOFEEDBACK

To locate a licensed clinician, contact:

Association for Applied Psychophysiology and Biofeedback
Wheat Ridge, CO; (800) 477-8892

ALCOHOLISM REHABILITATION

For referral to a therapist or support group, contact:

Alcoholics Anonymous (AA) World Service
New York, NY; (212) 870-3400

Al-Anon Family Group Headquarters
New York, NY; (800) 356-9996

SUBSTANCE ABUSE REHABILITATION

For referral to a therapist or support group, contact:

Drug-Anon Focus (a Division of Alcoholics Anonymous
World Service)
New York, NY; (212) 484-9095

National Association on Drug Abuse Problems
New York, NY; (212) 986-1170

SEX THERAPY OR COUPLES COUNSELING

For referral to a licensed therapist, contact:

American Association of Sex Educators, Counselors, and
Therapists (AASECT)
Chicago, IL; (312) 644-0828

Sex Information and Education Council of the US (SIECUS)
New York, NY; (212) 819-9770

STUDY OF MEN'S ISSUES

American Men's Studies Association
Northampton, MA; (413) 584-8903

PHYSICIANS PARTICIPATING IN ADVANCES IN MEDICINE
TO PROMOTE LONGEVITY

For a referral, contact:

American Academy of Anti-Aging Medicine
Chicago, IL; (773) 528-8500

Ahmed, S. R., A. E. Boucher, A. Manni, R. J. Santen, M. Bartholomew, and L. M. Demers. "Transdermal Testosterone Therapy in the Treatment of Male Hypogonadism." *Journal of Clinical Endocrinology and Metabolism* 66, no. 3 (March 1988): 546–51.

Akkus, E., S. Carrier, K. Baba, G. L. Hsu, H. Padma-Nathan, L. Nunes, and T. F. Lue. "Structural Alterations in The Tunica Albuginea of the Penis: Impact of Peyronie's Disease, Ageing, and Impotence." *British Journal of Urology* 79, no. 1 (January 1997): 47–53.

Anderson, R. A., J. Bancroft, and F. C. Wu. "The Effects of Exogenous Testosterone on Sexuality and Mood of Normal Men." *Journal of Clinical Endocrinology and Metabolism* 75, no. 6 (December 1992): 1503–7.

Bagatell, C. J., J. R. Heiman, A. M. Matsumoto, J. E. Rivier, and W. J. Bremner. "Metabolic and Behavioral Effects of High-Dose, Exogenous Testosterone in Healthy Men." *Journal of Clinical Endocrinology and Metabolism* 79, no. 2 (August 1994): 561–67.

Bals-Pratsch, M., U. A. Knuth, Y. D. Yoon, and E. Nieschlag. "Transdermal Testosterone Substitution Therapy for Male Hypogonadism." *Lancet* 2, no. 8513 (October 1986): 943–46.

Bals-Pratsch, M., K. Langer, V. A. Place, and E. Nieschlag. "Substitution Therapy of Hypogonadal Men with Transdermal Testosterone over One Year." *Acta Endocrinologica (Copenhagen)* 118, no. 1 (May 1988): 7–13.

Barrett-Connor, E., K. T. Khaw, and S. S. Yen. "Endogenous Sex Hormone Levels in Older Adult Men with Diabetes Mellitus." *American Journal of Epidemiology* 132, no. 5 (November 1990): 895–901.

Behre, H. M., S. Kliesch, E. Leifke, T. M. Link, and E. Nieschlag. "Long-Term Effect of Testosterone Therapy on Bone Mineral Density in Hypogonadal Men." *Journal of Clinical Endocrinology and Metabolism* 82, no. 8 (August 1997): 2386–90.

Berlin, F. S., and C. F. Meineke. "Treatment of Sex Offenders with Andiandrogenic Medication: Concept Valuation, Review of Treatment Modalities, and Preliminary Findings." *American Journal of Psychiatry* (1981): 138; 601–7.

Braverman, E. *PATH Wellness Manual*. Princeton, N.J.: Publications for Achieving Total Health, 1995.

Braverman, E., C. Pfeiffer, K. Blum, and R. Smayda. *The Healing Nutrients Within*. 2d ed. Los Angeles: Keats Publishing, 1997.

Brock, G., L. Nunes, H. Padma-Nathan, S. Boyd, and T. F. Lue. "Nitric Oxide Synthase: A New Diagnostic Tool for Neurogenic Impotence." *Urology* 42, no. 4 (October 1993): 412–17.

Brodsky, I. G., P. Balagopal, and K. S. Nair. "Effects of Testosterone Replacement on Muscle Mass and Muscle Protein Synthesis in Hypogonadal Men: A Clinical Research Study." *Journal of Clinical Endocrinology and Metabolism* 81, no. 10 (October 1996): 3469–75.

Casdorph, R., and M. Walker. *Toxic Metal Syndrome*. Garden City Park, N.Y.: Avery Publishing Group, 1995.

Cohen, A. S., R. C. Rosen, and L. Goldstein. "EEG hemispheric Asymmetry during Sexual Arousal: Psychophysiological Patterns in Responsive, Unresponsive, and Dysfunctional Men." *Journal of Abnormal Psychology* 94, no. 4 (1985): 580–90.

Cooper, T. G., C. Keck, U. Oberdieck, and E. Nieschlag. "Effects of Multiple Ejaculations after Extended Periods of Sexual Abstinence on Total, Motile, and Normal Sperm Numbers, As Well As Accessory Gland Secretions, from Healthy Normal and Oligozoospermic Men." *Human Reproduction* 8, no. 8 (1993): 1251–58.

Davidson, J. M., C. A. Camargo, and E. R. Smith. "Effects of Androgen on Sexual Behavior in Hypogonadal Men." *Journal of Clinical Endocrinology and Metabolism* 48, no. 6 (June 1979): 955–58.

de Lange, W. E., M. C. Snoep, H. Doorenbos. "The Effect of Short-Term Testosterone Treatment in Boys with Delayed Puberty." *Acta Endocrinologica (Copenhagen)* 91, no. 1 (May 1979): 177–83.

Finkelstein, J. W., E. J. Susman, V. M. Chinchilli, S. J. Kunselman, M. R. D'Arcangelo, J. Schwab, L. M. Demers, L. S. Liben, G. Lookingbill, and H. E. Kulin. "Estrogen or Testosterone Increases Self-Reported Aggressive Behaviors in Hypogonadal Adolescents." *Journal of Clinical Endocrinology and Metabolism* 82, no. 8 (August 1997): 2433–38.

Handa, K., H. Ishii, S. Kono, K. Shinchi, K. Imanishi, H. Mihara, and K. Tanaka. "Behavioral Correlates of Plasma Sex Hormones and Their Relationships with Plasma Lipids and Lipoproteins in Japanese Men." *Atherosclerosis* 130, no. 1–2 (April 1997): 37–44.

Haffner, S. M., J. Shaten, M. P. Stern, G. D. Smith, and L. Kuller. "Low Levels of Sex Hormone-Binding Globulin and Testosterone Predict the Development of Non-Insulin-Dependent Diabetes Mellitus in Men." *American Journal of Epidemiology* 143, no. 9 (May 1996): 889–97.

Hanlon, T. "Do You Need the Hormone of Desire." *Prevention* (August 1997): 73–79.

Hoffman, D. M., A. J. O'Sullivan, R. C. Baxter, and K. K. Ho. "Diagnosis of Growth-hormone Deficiency in Adults." *Lancet* 343, no. 8905 (April 1994): 1064–68.

Kaiser, F. E., "Sexuality and Impotence in the Aging Man." *Clinics in Geriatric Medicine* 7, no. 1 (February 1991): 63–72.

Katznelson, L., J. S. Finklestein, D. A. Schoenfeld, D. I. Rosenthal, E. J. Anderson, and A. Klibanski. "Increase in Bone Density and Lean Body Mass during Testosterone Administration in Men with Acquired Hypogonadism." *Journal of Clinical Endocrinology and Metabolism* 81, no. 12 (December 1996): 4358–65.

Kim, E. D., R. El-Rashidy, and K. T. McVary. "Papaverine Topical Gel for Treatment of Erectile Dysfunction." *Journal of Urology* 153, no. 2 (February 1995): 361–65.

Klatz, R., and C. Kahn. *Grow Young with HGH.* New York: HarperCollins, 1997.

Korenman, S. G., S. Viosca, D. Garza, M. Guralnik, V. Place, P. Campbell, and S. S. Davis. "Androgen Therapy of Hypogonadal Men with Transscrotal Testosterone Systems." *American Journal of Medicine* 83, no. 3 (September 1987): 471–78.

Luboshitzky R., P. Herer, and P. Lavie. "Pulsatile Patterns of Melatonin Secretion in Patients with Gonadotropin-Releasing Hormone Deficiency: Effects of Testosterone Replacement." *Journal of Pineal Research* 22, no. 2 (March 1997): 95–101.

Marin, P. "Testosterone and Regional Fat Distribution." *Obesity Research* Suppl. 4 (November 1995): 609S–612S.

Marin, P., H. Kvist, G. Lindstedt, L. Sjorstrom, and P. Bjorntorp. "Low Concentrations of Insulin-Like Growth Factor-1 in Abdominal Obesity." *International Journal of Obesity and Related Metabolic Disorders* 17, no. 2 (February 1993): 83–89.

McGivern, R. F., R. Z. Sokol, and W. R. Adey. "Prenatal Exposure to a Low-Frequency Electromagnetic Field Demasculinizes Adult Scent Marking Behavior and Increases Accessory Sex Organ Weights in Rats." *Tetralogy* 41, no. 1 (January 1990): 1–8.

Mikhailichenko, V. V., O. L. Tiktinskii, P. A. Sil'nitskii, N. V. Vorokhombina, and V. P. Aleksadrov. "The Pathogenesis of Sexual Disorders in Men with Diabetes Mellitus." *Urologiia I Nefrologiia (Moskva)* 2 (March 1993): 47–50.

Moller, J. *Cholesterol.* New York: Springer-Verlag, 1987.

Money, J. "Treatment Guidelines: Anti-androgen and Counseling of Paraphilic Sex Offenders." *Journal of Sex and Marital Therapy* 13, no. 3 (1987): 219–23.

Montague, D. *Disorders of Male Sexual Function.* Chicago: YearBook Medical Publishers, Inc., 1988.

Morales, A. J., J. J. Nolan, J. C. Nelson, and S. S. Yen. "Effects of Replacement Dose of Dehydroepiandrosterone in Men and Women of Advancing Age." *Journal of Clinical Endocrinology and Metabolism* 78, no. 6 (June 1994): 1360–67.

Murray, F. T., H. U. Wyss, R. G. Thomas, M. Spevack, and A. G. Glaros. "Gonadal Dysfunction in Diabetic Men with Organic Impotence." *Journal of Clinical Endocrinology and Metabolism* 65, no. 1 (July 1987): 127–35.

Padma-Nathan, H., S. D. Boyd, and D. Cheung. "The Biochemical Effect of Aging, Diabetes, and Ischaemia on Corporal and Tunical Collagen." *Journal of Urology* 145 (1991): 324A.

Padma-Nathan, H., W. J. Hellstrom, F. E. Kaiser, R. F. Labasky, T. F. Lue , W. E. Nolten, P. C. Norwood, C. A. Peterson, R. Shabsigh, and P. Y. Tam. "Treatment of Men with Erectile Dysfunction with Transurethral Alprostadil: Medicated Urethral System for Erection (MUSE) Study Group." *New England Journal of Medicine* 336, no. 1 (January 1997): 1–7.

Pfeiffer, C. *Zinc and Other Micro-Nutrients.* Los Angeles: Keats Publishing, 1978.

Pfeilschifter, J., C. Scheidt-Nave, G. Leidig-Bruckner, H. W. Woitge, W. F. Blum, C. Wuster, D. Haack, and R. Ziegler. "Relationship between Circulating Insulin-Like Growth Factor Components and Sex Hormones in a Population-based Sample of 50- to 80-year-old Men and Women."*Journal of Clinical Endocrinology and Metabolism* 81, no. 7 (July 1996): 2534–40.

Phillips, G. B. "Relationship Between Serum Sex Hormones and the Glucose-Insulin-Lipid Defect in Men with Obesity." *Metabolism* 42, no. 1 (January 1993): 116–20.

Phillips, G. B., T. Y. Jing, L. M. Resnick, M. Barbagllo, J. H. Laragh, and J. E. Sealey. "Sex Hormones and Hemostatic Risk Factors for Coronary Heart Disease in Men with Hypertension." *Journal of Hypertension* 11, no. 7 (July 1993): 699–702.

Phillips, G. B., B. H. Pinkernell, and T. Y. Jing. "The Association of Hypotestosteronemia with Coronary Artery Disease in Men." *Arteriosclerosis and Thrombosis* 14, no. 5 (May 1994): 701–6.

Pierpaoli, W., and W. Regelson. *The Melatonin Miracle.* New York: Simon & Schuster, 1995.

Ponjee, G. A., H. A. De Rooy, and H. L. Vander. "Androgen Turnover during Marathon Running." *Medicine and Science in Sports Exercise* 26, no. 10 (October 1994): 1274–77.

Renganathan, R., B. Suranjan, and T. Kurien. "Comparison of Transdermal Nitroglycerin and Intracavernous Injection of Papaverine in the Treatment of Erectile Dysfunction in Patients with Spinal Cord Lesions." *Spinal Cord* 35, no. 2 (February 1997): 99–103.

Rosen, R. C., and J. G. Beck. *Patterns of Sexual Arousal: Psychophysiological Processes and Clinical Applications.* New York: The Guilford Press, 1988.

Schiavi, R., and J. Rehman. "Sexuality and Aging." *Urologic Clinics of North America* 22, no. 4 (1995).

Segal, K. R., A. Dunaif, B. Gutin, J. Albu, A. Nyman, and F. X. Pi-Sunyer. "Body Composition, Not Body Weight, Is Related to Cardiovascular Disease Risk Factors and Sex Hormone Levels in Men." *Journal of Clinical Investigation* 80, no. 4 (October 1987): 1050–55.

Shealy, C. Norman, M.D., Ph.D. *DHEA: The Youth and Health Hormone.* Los Angeles: Keats Publishing, 1996.

Sih, R., J. E. Morley, F. E. Kaiser, H. M. Perry III, P. Patrick, and C. Ross. "Testosterone Replacement in Older Hypogonadal Men: A 12-month Randomized Controlled Trial." *Journal of Clinical Endocrinology and Metabolism* 82, no. 6 (June 1997): 1661–67.

Sonksen, J., and F. Biering-Sorensen. "Transcutaneous Nitroglycerin in the Treatment of Erectile Dysfunction in Spinal Cord Injured." *Paraplegia* 30, no. 8 (August 1992): 554–57.

Tang, S. F., N. K. Chu, and M. K. Wong. "Intracavernous Injection of Prostaglandin E1 in Spinal Cord Injured Patients with Erectile Dysfunction: A Preliminary Report." *Paraplegia* 33, no. 12 (December 1995): 731–33.

Tenover, J. S. "Effects of Testosterone Supplementation in the Aging Male." *Journal of Clinical Endocrinology and Metabolism* 75, no. 4 (October 1992): 1092–98.

Uyanik, B. S., Z. Ari, B. Gumus, M. R. Yigitoglu, and T. Arslan. "Beneficial Effects of Testosterone Undecanoate on the Lipoprotein Profiles in Health Elderly Men: A Placebo Controlled Study." *Japanese Heart Journal* 38, no. 1 (January 1997): 73–82.

Wang, C., G. Alexander, N. Berman, B. Salehian, T. Davidson, V. McDonald, B. Steiner, L. Hull, C. Callegari, and R. S. Swerdloff. "Testosterone Replacement Therapy Improves Mood in Hypogonadal Men: A Clinical Research Center Study." *Journal of Clinical Endocrinology and Metabolism* 81, no. 10 (October 1996): 3578–83.

Wincze, J. P., S. Bansal, and M. Malamud. "Effects of Medroxyprogesterone Acetate on Subjective Arousal, Arousal to Erotic Stimulation, and Nocturnal Penile Tumescence in Male Sex Offenders." *Archives of Sexual Behavior* 15, no. 4 (August 1986): 293–305.

Vermeulen, A. "The Male Climacterium." *Annals of Medicine* 25, no. 6 (December 1993): 531–34.

Zacharin, M. R., and G. L. Warne. "Treatment of Hypogonadal Adolescent Boys with Long-Acting Subcutaneous Testosterone Pellets." *Archives of Disease in Childhood* 76, no. 6 (June 1997): 495–99.

Zilbergeld, B. *The New Male Sexuality.* New York: Bantam Books, 1992.